Balance Exercises for Fall Prevention

Step By Step Guide To Balance Exercises For Seniors Over 40 And Everyone

D1410198

Introduction

If you have ever fallen—it does not matter how old you were—, you know how embarrassing it can be, especially if you fell in front of people. You probably got lucky and didn't get injured, had minor injuries like bruises, strains, or sprains, or had serious injuries that affected your ability to do day-to-day activities on your own, e.g., broken or dislocated bones.

Well, if you have never fallen, don't be so proud of yourself yet. Do you know why? Your chances of falling increase day by day since our muscles lose strength and reflexes slow down as you age.

According to the Centers for Disease Control and Prevention, more than 1 out of 4 seniors fall every year, and 3 million of them are taken to hospitals for fall injuries. But guess what, you won't be one of them because you came to the right place.

This book will provide you with the best guide to balance exercises for seniors over 40 and everyone, hence preventing loss of mobility and independence or even death resulting from falls.

Let's begin your journey to leading a "fall-free" life!

PS: I'd like your feedback. If you are happy with this book, please leave a review on Amazon.

Please leave a review for this book on Amazon by visiting the page below:

https://amzn.to/2VMR5qr

Table of Contents

Chapter 4: Cool-down Exercise/Stretches 83

Chapter 1: Muscles Associated With Balance and Stability

Sometimes, when you are sitting or standing, you might feel unsteady, dizzy, or light-headed, and your body might feel as if it is moving, floating, or spinning, an experience that can make you fall. This can happen to anyone at any age and can result from weak muscles.

This chapter focuses on the three main muscles, i.e., the core muscles, the glute muscles, and the erector spinae muscles) that give you balance and stability. We will mainly be looking at their location, how they function to prevent falls and the benefits of exercising/strengthening them (with the main one being fall prevention).

Core Muscles

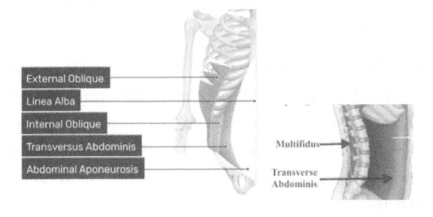

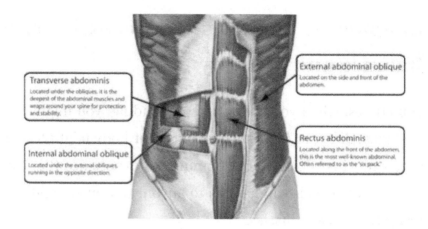

Core muscles are all the body muscles that connect to the spine and the pelvic. The major core muscles are the rectus abdominis muscles, internal and external oblique, erector spinae muscles, transverse abdominis, and multifidus.

The Rectus Abdominis Muscles

Also called "The abs," the rectus abdominis muscles are 2 long pairs of muscles found at the sides of the abdomen walls (each side with one pair). They connect the pelvis and the ribs using linea alba tissues.

It is important to have strong rectus abdominis muscles because they are responsible for moving the trunk forward, sideways, and back, stabilizing the spine, and pelvis movements, which affects posture. These muscles also help in breathing, i.e., exhalation, as they pull down the breathing muscles.

Internal Oblique Muscles

The internal oblique is a broad and thin lateral muscle found on the abdominal sides. It originates from the anterior iliac crest and the inguinal ligament and inserts on the linea alba, the abdominal aponeurosis, and the cartilages of the 4 lower ribs.

Unilaterally (one-side), internal oblique muscles help rotate and laterally flex the torso to the same side, and bilaterally (both sides) help in the flexion and compression of the trunk and its contents. Together with other abdominal wall muscles, it helps maintain normal tension in the abdominal wall.

External Oblique Muscles

The external oblique is the largest and primary muscle of the three abdominal wall muscles found on both the body's left and right sides. This muscle originates from the 8 lower ribs and inserts into the pubic bone, the iliac crest, the abdominal aponeurosis, and the linea alba.

Unilaterally, external oblique muscles help rotate and laterally flex the torso to the opposite side. Also, this muscle helps flex and compress the trunk and its contents bilaterally.

Transverse Abdominis Muscles

Found under internal oblique muscles, transverse abdominis muscles are a thin and flat sheet of muscles. They arise from the anterior iliac crest, the thoracolumbar fascia, the 6 lower ribs, the iliac fascia, and the inguinal ligament and insert into the symphysis pubis, the xiphoid process, and the linea alba.

Together with other abdominal muscles, the transverse abdominis muscle helps increase pressure in the intraabdominal, which helps in forceful experiences such as coughing, urinating, defecation, and expiration. These muscles also help stabilize the pelvis and the lumbar spine before and during limb movements.

Multifidus Muscles

Multifidus muscles are the second extensor back muscles layer located at the left and right sides of the spinal column.

It compromises a series of small and triangular muscles. These muscles originate from the transverse processes (of the vertebrae) at the lumbar, the sacrum, the thoracic, and the cervical regions and insert into the spinous processes.

The function of the multifidus muscles (together with other deep back muscles) is to help with arch movements of the back and help the abdominal muscles in the tilting and twisting of the body. In other words, when they contract unilaterally, they result in side rotation and bending, and when they contract bilaterally, they extend the back.

Also, due to the unique design that gives them strength, multifidus muscles help stabilize the vertebrae during spinal movements.

Advantages of Strengthening Your Core Muscles

Working out to strengthen your core will give you balance and stability hence preventing falls and injuries. You will be able to do any movements, e.g., sitting, standing, twisting, bending, and rotating, without the fear of falling but, do you know what more benefits you will get from exercising your core muscles?

- **Improved posture:** Whether or not you are a senior, it is important to have a good posture because good posture prevents spinal wear and tear. It also helps boost confidence in your daily encounter and allows you to breathe deeply due to increased intraabdominal pressure.

- **It makes daily activities bearable:** Almost all daily activities depend on your core muscles; hence, strengthening them through exercises will make it easier to perform actions such as sitting, standing, bending, twisting, overhead reaching, lifting, and carrying.

- **Improves performance in pleasurable activities and hobbies or sports:** If you enjoy fun activities such as golfing, swimming or tennis, a strong core will enable you to perform them to surprisingly old age. Also, working on your core muscles will improve your flexibility and core strength, which is important during sex.

- **Helps prevent or reduce pain:** A strong core translates to reduced lower back and spine pain because it helps mitigate and avoid discomforts and irritations from behaviors such as sitting, standing, and bending.

- **Abs and slim waistline:** By exercising your core, you will be able to walk proudly at the beach with a bare chest or a bikini because exercises for strengthening the core lead to a reduced waistline and the development of "six-pack abs."

Now that you have a brief knowledge of the core muscles, let's look at another group of muscles that can lead to imbalance when not exercised and well taken care of:

Glute Muscles

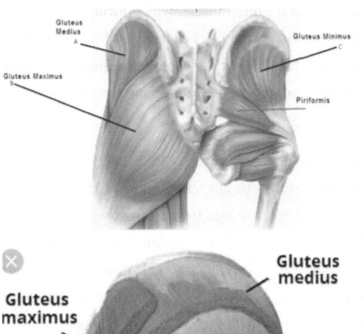

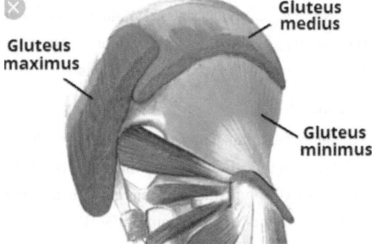

The glute muscles —also called the butt muscles— are found on the buttocks and play a big role in maintaining body balance. These muscles include:

Gluteus Maximus

This is the biggest glute muscle, which forms most buttocks. Gluteus maximus is one of the strongest body muscles that originate from the sides of the coccyx, the ilium, the sacrum's lower parts, and the aponeurosis and inserts into gluteal tuberose and fascia late.

Together with other glute muscles, the gluteus Maximus helps in hip extension, lateral rotation of the hip, and hip abduction, allowing the legs to move backward and forward. This muscle acts to maintain balance during actions that require force, e.g., climbing stairs, standing from a sitting position, running, bending, and straightening. The Gluteus maximus also supports the trunk and the pelvis.

Gluteus Medius

As the name suggests, the gluteus medius is the middle glute muscle found underneath the gluteus maximus. It originates from the ilium (the hipbone) and inserts into the greater trochanter of the femur (on the lateral surface).

Like the gluteus maximus, the gluteus medius plays a role in the lateral hip rotation, abduction, and medial rotation. It also helps maintain pelvis stability during movement, e.g., Climbing the stairs and walking.

Gluteus Minimus

This is the smallest glute muscle. It originates from the ilium and inserts into the greater trochanter of the femur (on the anterior surface).

The Gluteus minimus helps stabilize the pelvis and the hip when you are standing on both or one leg, walking or running. It also uses its anterior part to rotate the thigh internally and its posterior part to rotate the thigh externally.

Benefits of Exercising the Glute Muscles

Nowadays, most people spend more time sitting, i.e., at work and home, than they do standing. This means the butt muscles get used too much and become weak (i.e., underactive and overstretched). The hip flexors become tight and overactive; hence, they stop working as strongly and effectively as expected. That is why you need to create time to do some workouts that target your glute muscles.

Some of the benefits of exercising your glute muscles are:

Pain and Injury Prevention

Glute muscles work together in hip abduction, flexion, and extension. When these muscles are weak, your body loses balance, making simple activities such as running and climbing difficult, a condition that can easily make you fall.

Also, since weak glute muscles cannot perform their main role, having too tight or overstretched glute muscles forces the body to look for other body muscles to do the hip abduction and hip extension role (which is not their role). This can make the helping muscles overstressed and overused, leading to imbalance and pain in the hips, knees, and spine. Exercising the glute muscles will prevent all these from happening by improving your balance on your hip and pelvic areas and making them strong for their role.

Improved Athletic and Exercise Performance

Strong glute muscles will improve your balance, prevent injuries, and give you the best results in athletic if you are an athlete or interested in joining sporting activities. This is because your glute muscles are the ones that enable or will enable you to speed up, slow down, change direction and give you the power to jump. So if you are into sporting activities such as cycling, jumping, and running, exercising your glute muscles will give your hips the power to push your body forward.

Also, working out your glute muscles will make it easier to perform other body parts' exercises that require the strength of your glute and hips, e.g., press-ups.

Improved Posture

Weak glute muscles, i.e., overstretched hip extensors or underdeveloped glutes, i.e., short and tight thigh flexors, can lead to poor posture, affecting your stability since the glute muscles are responsible for your ability to stand up.

However, exercising your glute muscles will help stabilize your body and strengthen your back, which will help you avoid slouching. Also, training your glute muscles will prevent your belly from "pooching"- a condition where weak or too tight hips tilt forward, causing the abdomen to move out (even when you do not have belly fat).

Also, the glute muscles work together with the core muscles to support and stabilize the spine, making it possible to move, sit, or stand.

Prevention or Reduction of Knee Pain

Your lower body muscles work as a group. That is why an unstable hip can lead to excessive medial rotation (where the femur moves inwards), leading to a condition known as lateral patellar tracking (where the kneecaps move out of place when you straighten or bend your leg). Exercising your glute muscles will improve your pelvis and hip stability hence avoiding discomfort or pain on the knees.

Ability to Do Your Daily Tasks

Sara Lewis, a celebrity trainer who created XO Fitness in Los Angeles, says that all body muscles work as expected when we have strong glute muscles, making it easier to go about daily activities. This is because the glute muscles connect the upper body and the lower body; hence, the stronger the muscles, the stronger the connection and the better the performance.

Also, strengthening your glute muscles will reduce or relieve back pain (a problem most people experience during daily activities) because all your back muscles rely on the glute muscles.

From there, let's get to the last group of muscles that play a big role in ensuring your stability and balance.

Erector Muscles

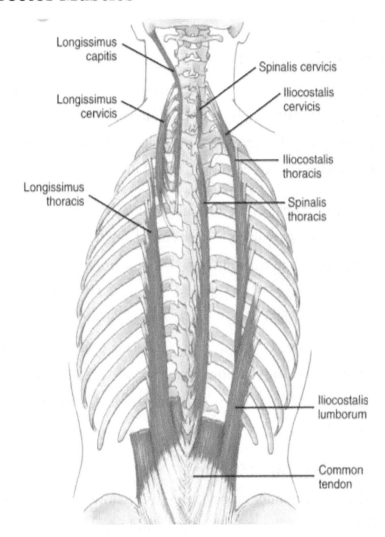

Longissimus capitis

Longissimus cervicis

Longissimus thoracis

Spinalis cervicis

Iliocostalis cervicis

Iliocostalis thoracis

Spinalis thoracis

Iliocostalis lumborum

Common tendon

Also known as the extensor spinae or the sacrospinalis, the erector spinae is a group of muscles found on both the left and right sides of the spine/vertebral column, starting from the hips and the sacrum, extending up through the thoracic region and into the cervix. The erector spinae muscles have three main groups. i.e.

The Spinalis Muscle

The spinalis muscle is the deepest, smallest and medial erector spinae muscle. It is subdivided into 3, i.e., spinalis capitis, spinalis thoracis, and spinalis cervicis, which joins the spinous process of vertebrae together.

The spinalis capitis origin and insertion is by way of blending with semispinalis capitis. The spinalis cervicis originates from the ligament nuchal, the spinous process of C7 (the seventh cervical vertebra) and sometimes T1 to T2 (the 1st and the 2nd thoracic vertebra), and inserts into the spinous processes of the C2, C3, and C4. The spinalis thoracis originates from the spinous process of T11 and L2 (the second lumbar spinae vertebra) and inserts into the upper thoracic vertebra.

The Longissimus Muscle

Lateral to the spinalis muscle, the longissimus muscle is the middle muscle of the erector spinae and forms the meat part of this muscle group.

The longissimus muscle usually attaches to the vertebral transverse process and is divided into 3, i.e., the longissimus capitis, longissimus cervicis, and longissimus thoracis.

The longissimus capitis originates from the transverse process of C4 to T4 and inserts into the mastoid process (on its posterior edge). The longissimus cervicis originates from T1 to T4 and inserts into the transverse process of C2 to C6. The longissimus thoracis originates from the lumbar vertebrae's transverse processes and sometimes blends the iliocostalis (the third erector spinae muscle). It inserts into the transverse processes of the thoracic region.

The Illiocostalis Muscle

This is the most lateral erector spinae muscle that attaches to the ribs. Like the other erector spinae muscles, it is divided into 3, i.e., iliocostalis cervicis, iliocostalis thoracis, and iliocostalis lumborum.

The iliocostalis cervicis originates from the third to the sixth upper ribs and inserts into the transverse process of C4 to C6, while the iliocostalis thoracis originates from the 6 lower ribs and inserts into the transverse process of C7 and the 6 upper ribs.

The iliocostalis lumborum originates from the iliac crest and inserts into the thoracolumbar fascia, the transverse processes of L1 to L4, and the 4th to 12th upper ribs.

Bilaterally, all the erector spinae muscles work together to keep the spine in its natural curvature, giving you an upright posture. They are also responsible for back extension (the ability to bend backward), lateral back rotation (the ability to twist your back on each side and look behind you), lateral back flexion (the ability to side bend), and the unilateral rotation of the head.

Benefits of Strong Erector Spinae and the Entire Back Muscles

The erector spinae muscles do not work alone, and most back exercises you will perform target most (if not all) of your back muscles, which is why we shall look at the remarkable results you will get from all the back exercises.

Below are some of them:

Upright Posture Hence Improved Balance

As we age, we tend to lean forward, but this is not always the case for people who have included some back exercise sessions in their workout routine.

Back exercises improve your posture by keeping your erector spinae muscles strong, which in turn keeps the spine erect. Neglecting to exercise your back muscles will lead to poor posture, which causes imbalanced shoulders. Shoulder imbalance can affect your stability, making it easier to fall.

Improved Sex Life

Studies have shown that people who do regular back exercises can have lasting and better sex experiences than those who do not. This is because back exercises improve lower back movement and reduce the chances of erectile dysfunction in men. Also, back exercises help reduce or prevent lower back pain; lower back pain is a known hindrance to a healthy sex life.

Strengthens and Protects Your Spine

Without your spine, you would be someone who relies on other people for survival because your spine is responsible for your locomotive activities and your nervous system. That is why you need to relieve stress and pressure from your spinal code and make it strong through back exercises, especially those that target the erector spinae muscles.

Think of it this way, even when you slip and fall, the chances of spinal injuries after starting your workout routine will be lower than if you fell now (when your back muscles and the spine are not as strong as they can be) because your spinal cord will have a strong armor.

However, doing back exercises will require you to be cautious by performing every move correctly. This is because incorrectly performed back exercises can lead to spine injuries.

Improved Overall Well-being

Back exercises improve blood circulation in the body, which results in faster transmission of nutrients to different body parts. This means if you do back exercises regularly, you will always be full of energy and will have the general body strength to do your daily tasks (even the high-intensity ones).

Also, you will have improved neurotransmission; hence, you will experience many benefits such as reduced stress, fatigue, and depression.

If you dream of having an admirable, coveted and nice V-shaped back, regular back exercises will help you with balance and make your upper body shape dreams come true.

Now that you know some anatomy of the main muscles responsible for balance, how they work, and why you need them to work as they should, you should know one thing:

Although this book focuses on exercises that target the involved muscles, we shall also look into full-body exercises because, as mentioned earlier, all muscles work together. Therefore, working out some muscles while neglecting others won't give you the best results possible.

Let's get to the interesting part you have been waiting for!

Chapter 2: Warm Up Exercises

If you are wondering why you need warm-up exercises when you can get right into balance exercises, here is why.

At the start of any workout session, you need around 5-10 minutes to prepare your body, muscles, and mind for the main exercise to get optimal results at the end of the session.

When reading an article, you have to start from the beginning to the main part and then to the end. Similarly, working out has a beginning too, i.e., warm-up exercises.

These exercises include slow-paced, low-intensity activities that warm up your muscles by increasing your temperatures, making the muscles ready for the strenuous moves that will follow.

It is very tempting to jump right into the main exercise but don't; if you do, you won't get the best results as your body, brain, and muscles might take up to 10 minutes before they are ready to do the exercise well, and you might end up causing more harm than good.

 Let's look at other benefits of warming up:

Benefits of Warm-Up Exercises

Some of the benefits you will get from taking time to warm up before every workout session are:

Increased muscle and body temperature

Warm-up exercises increase muscle and body temperature, improving blood flow in body tissues. Increased blood flow to tissues leads to an increase in the availability of oxygen in the muscles, making them relax and contract with ease during the main exercise, ensuring they don't get torn or strained. Also, improved blood flow enhances the delivery of nutrients in the body hence boosting energy levels.

Performing some warm-ups will also give your heart time to prepare to pump blood faster during your balance exercise sessions, which will help you avoid straining it.

Lower Risk of Injury

Warm-ups will make your body flexible and muscles more elastic, meaning you will be able to maintain or regain your balance without hurting yourself or having cases of overheating.

These exercises give the body time to change from the activities it was doing, thereby helping it prepare for the main exercises, which might be intense.

Also, the communication between the nervous system and the muscles will improve, which will make your body respond faster to new moves; hence, you will be able to introduce new and challenging exercises safely and efficiently.

Warm-up workouts also slow down the production of lactic acid, which makes the body feel sore and tired when built up in the muscles. Lower lactic acid levels allow you to exercise for the required time and endure vigorous exercises without the risk of injuring your muscles.

Mental Preparedness

Doing some warm-up will help you separate your workout session thoughts from other thoughts by bringing your concentration to the present. The workouts will give you some time to clear your mind, put aside any stress or worries, and increase your on the task at hand, thereby increasing your primary exercise performance.

Motivation

Some days you might feel lazy and want to skip your workout sessions; on some other days, when the going gets tough, you might want to quit. But even during these days, put on your workout clothes and start doing your warm-up exercises.

The chances are high that you will feel ready and willing to continue your balance exercises after warming up. If you are recovering from an illness or an injury, your experience from your warm-up exercises will help you know if you are ready for the main exercises or not.

Activates Your Joints and Core

Warming up will make your joints mobile and increase their flexibility, leading to an increase in power and efficiency and the prevention of joint injuries during your main session. Warming up your spine, core, back, and glute muscles will allow you to control your movements by preparing your body to maintain balance and stability

All the above benefits aim at making your balance workout sessions successful.

EffectiveWarm-Up Exercises

Let us look at some warm-up exercises you can try:

Bird Dog Exercise

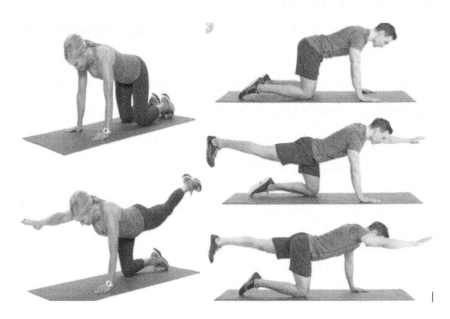

This easy-to-do exercise targets and activates the glute, lower back, core muscles, and hip flexor. Bird dog is suitable for anyone (unless advised otherwise by your doctor), and the only things you need are a yoga mat or a cushioned surface and a spot where you can extend one leg and one arm simultaneously.

- Start in an all four position, with your arms at shoulder width and your knees at hip-width. Push your shoulder blades backward, tighten your abs, and let your spine take its natural curvature.

- Raise and straighten your right hand in front of you and extend your left leg backward until they both are in a straight line and parallel or almost parallel (depending on how high you can go) to the ground. Keep your shoulders and head straight and aligned. If your low back starts to sag, you can lift your leg slightly higher to maintain a straight back.

- Stay in this position for a few seconds.

- Slowly return your hand and knee to the starting position.

- Switch to your left hand and right leg and perform the above moves.

- Do 10 repetitions on each side.

If you find it challenging to raise your leg and arm simultaneously, you can start with straightening one leg at a time with no arm raise or by raising them just an inch or two off the ground and then progress to the full range move when you feel firm.

The 90-90 Movement

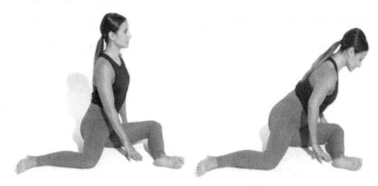

The 90-90 exercise increases hip mobility and activates the glute muscles through internal rotation of one hip and external rotation of the other.

How to do it

- Sit on your exercise mat and position your left leg before you, ensuring the hip rotates outward. Make sure the lower leg part is touching the ground, your ankle is neutral, and your leg is at a 90 degrees angle.

- Place your right leg behind you to rotate its hip outward. Bend your knee to a 90 degrees angle, keeping your ankle and sheen on the ground. Ensure that your hip and knee are in line and your ankle is neutral. This position should result with your shoulder and hip in line and your knee and your right hand (should you raise it straight).

- Sit tall and support your position by putting your left hand beside you, with your palm facing down and pointing backward.

- Lean forward by hovering over your left knee; do your best to resist the urge to tilt to one side.

- Actively push down your left knee and ankle for 5 seconds. You should feel a stretch on your hip or groin area.

- Slowly return to starting position and hold for 5 seconds. Remember to maintain an upright posture.

- Continue this movement for 60 seconds.

- Switch sides such that your right leg is in front and your left leg is behind you and repeat the above movement.

- Perform 3-4 reps on both sides.

If you find it challenging to stay upright, place a rolled-up towel or yoga block underneath the hip of the front leg. However, if you experience a sharp pain in any part of your body, slowly release your position and try another warm-up exercise.

Jumping Jacks Exercise

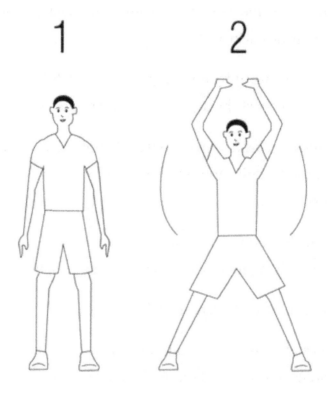

Jumping jacks are a warm-up exercise that targets your lungs, heart, and muscles, specifically the glutes, hip flexors, abdominals, quadriceps, and shoulder muscles. Hence, it is a good preparation exercise.

How to do it

- Stand straight on your exercise mat with your hands on your sides.

- Jump up, spreading your legs apart (beyond hip-width), and raise your hand above your head to a touching or almost touching position.

- Jump again to return to starting position by bringing your feet together and lowering your hands.

- Continue for a minute or 2, jumping as fast as you can.

You can modify jumping jacks by doing rotational jacks or squat jacks.

For rotational jacks:

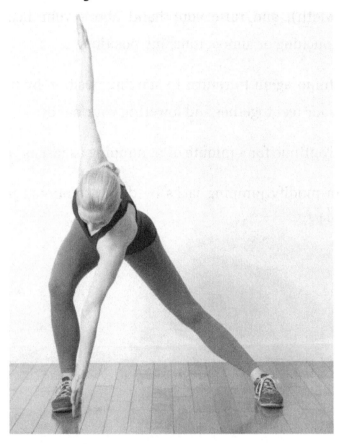

- Stand straight with your hands on your chest and your legs together.

- Jump up and land with your feet beyond your shoulder width and your toes pointing towards the out side.

- Bend your knees to assume a squatting position and rotation to your waist as your right hand reaches the ground, and the left hand reaches up.

- Jump up to return to your starting position.

- Repeat this movement on the other side such that your left hand will be on the floor and your right one will be pointing up to the sky.

- Continue this exercise, alternating sides for 10 -20 repetitions.

To perform squat jacks:

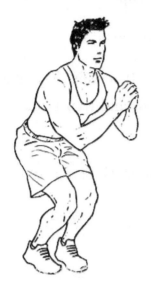 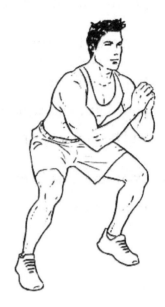

- Start by performing a few jumping jacks. Then, when your feet are apart, put your hands behind your ears or hold them together in front of the chest and get into a squat.

- Hold this position for a few seconds, then jump back to the standing position with hands still on your head or in front of you.

- Repeat the above moves for a minute or 2.

If you cannot jump, maybe because of an injury or age, you still can perform walking jacks or low impact jumping jacks through the following steps:

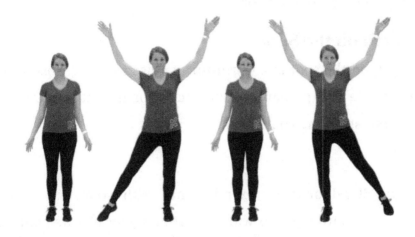

- Stand up straight and lift your hands over your head while stepping your right leg out.

- Return your hands and right leg to the starting position, immediately lift your hands over your head and take an outward step with your left leg.

- Return your hands and left leg to the starting position.

- Continue this movement for 30 seconds.

- Repeat the above moves, with your left side taking the lead for another 30 seconds.

When doing any of the above jacks, put on supportive shoes, e.g., sports sneakers, choose an even and flat space preferably with rubber, mat, or grass and, remember that speed is the key to having good results.

March on the Spot

March on the spot is a warm-up exercise that will raise your heart rate and prepare your muscles for the main exercises without straining your joints.

How to do it

- Stand on your exercise mat with your feet facing forward and hip-width apart and your elbows bent on your sides at an angle of 90 degrees.

- Lift your right knee such that your right thigh is parallel to the ground, and move your left elbow forward.

- Return your right leg and left hand to starting position.

- Bring your left knee up and move your right elbow forward.

- Return them to the starting position.

- Continue this exercise, alternating sides for a minute, all while trying to be as fast as possible.

Wall Angles

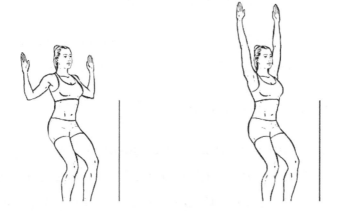

Wall angles warm up your thoracic spine, neck muscle, shoulder muscles, joints, and upper back muscles.

How to do it

- Stand on your mat with your back against the wall, arms on your sides and, legs at shoulder-width - 2-3 steps (6-10 inches) from the wall. Slightly bend your knee to make this position more comfortable.

- Get into a "hands up" pose by bending your elbows to a 90 degrees angle and raising your upper arm such that your shoulders and back of your palms and hands are on the wall.

- Engaging your core, lift your hands such that they form a "V" shape over your head but keep them against the wall. Try to raise your arms as high as possible, avoiding any urge to arch your back, protrude your neck or lift your hips.

- Slowly, push your shoulder blades down to return your arms and elbows to starting position.

- Perform 10- 15 repetitions.

If you find it uncomfortable to perform wall angles, you can switch to floor angles. Here, you will be performing all the wall angles steps but with your face-up on the floor and feet flat on the floor.

You can start your warm-up by performing single-arm wall or floor angles (where you raise one hand at a time and complete 1 rep after lifting each hand) for 10 reps, floor angles for 10 reps, and then wall angles for 15 reps.

Overhead Side Reach

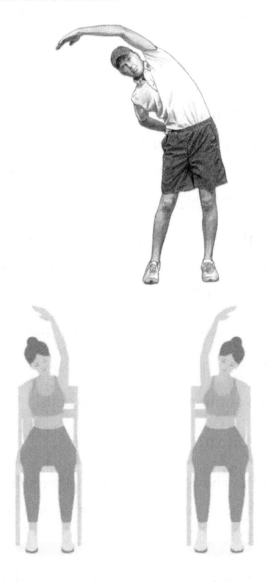

Overhead side reach is a warm-up that targets the obliques, shoulder, neck, and lower back muscles.

- Stand on your mat with your feet at shoulder width or further.

- Position your right hand on your waist and raise your left hand. Extend your shoulders and elbow such that your hand is over your head like you are reaching for something on the right side. Keep your fingers pointing to the sky.

- Lean to the right and lower your right hand slowly to your side until you feel a sudden power pull on the left side of your trunk.

- Relax your neck by letting it sink and drop to the stretch.

- Hold this position for about 30 seconds.

- Slowly return to the starting position.

- Repeat the above moves on the other side, i.e., with your left hand on your waist and your right hand overhead.

- Continue this exercise, alternating sides for 20 repetitions.

When doing this exercise, make sure to engage your core when leaning in to avoid injuring your spine. Also, let your neck relax and drop or adjust your lean whenever you feel any strain to avoid injuring it.

If this warm-up is too much, you can start by doing it while seated, or you can do it against a wall for support, then advance to standing on your own.

Other good warm-up exercises that can integrate well into your workout routine are jogging, cycling, walking, jumping rope, or swimming.

Now that you are warmed up, let's get to the exercises.

Chapter 3: Balance Exercises For Fall Prevention

Balance exercises involve moves that aim at strengthening the muscles that help keep you upright and stable, e.g., the core muscles, leg muscles, glute muscles, and back muscles.

These exercises can be both simple and intense; therefore, if you already have balance issues, start with the simple ones and advance to the intense ones with time. Below are some balance exercises you can try out:

Balance Exercises

Here are some of the best balance exercises:

Walking on a Straight Line Exercise

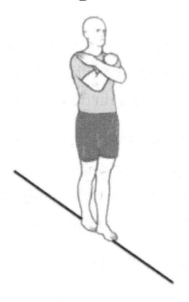

For this exercise, you need a hallway or an open space where you can draw a straight chalk line. You can also use existing straight lines, e.g., a flooring line in your hall.

How to do it

- Stand at one end of the straight line, put your arms on your waist, cross them on your chest, or stretch them out on your sides. Maintain an upright posture and keep your head looking forward.

- Walk on the line and every time you lift a foot, hold it for a second or two before moving it forward.

- Keep walking until you get to the other end of the line and try as much as possible to maintain balance by looking forward and keeping your focus on the line. If you have to look down, don't look at your feet. Instead, keep your gaze a few feet in front of you.

- When you get to the other end, you can walk backward without looking; you can also turn around by first bringing your feet together and slowly turning around, then walking back to the beginning end.

- Continue walking on the line for 10 minutes or so.

You can start by doing this exercise next to a wall for support in case you totter, but do not lean sideways or forward.

You can increase your stability by softening your knees and leaving small spaces between your feet when you take a step forward or backward. Keep a regular breathing pattern and move in a slow and steady motion.

Sumo Squat

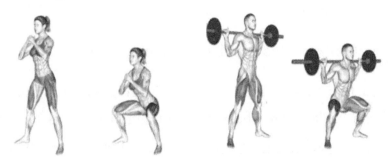

The Sumo squat exercise activates the hip abductor, core muscles, and leg muscles, improving balance and stability.

Until you are ready to challenge yourself, you will not need any equipment for this exercise. When you are ready to challenge yourself, you will need kettlebells, dumbbells, or barbells.

How to do it

- Stand on your mat with your feet wider than shoulder-width apart. Position your toes at about 45 degrees such that your hips rotate outward.

- Straighten your hands in front of you or hold them together in front of your chest, take a deep breath in, bend your knees forward and push your hips back to lower yourself into a squat. Maintain an upright back and a tight torso.

- Hold this position for 5 to 10 seconds.

- Exhale as you slowly push yourself up to the starting position.

- Continue this exercise for 10 minutes or so.

If you find this exercise a bit challenging, you can start by doing a basic squat where you do the above moves but with your toes facing forward and feet at shoulder width, then advance to sumo squat.

You can modify your sumo squats by reducing your speed or holding weights, e.g., 2kg dumbbells or an exercise ball. However, if you wish to add heavy dumbbells or barbells, work with a coach or a trainer to maintain proper posture.

You can also try sumo squat with outer thigh pulse through the following steps:

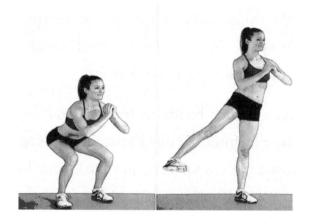

- Perform sumo squats for a few minutes.

- After standing from a squatting position, lift your left leg to the side. Keep your hands in the front or extend your right hand to the side. Lift your leg as high as you can.

- Hold for a few seconds, then return to the starting position.

- Repeat the above step with your right leg and left hand extended.

- Continue this exercise for 15 repetitions, alternating sides.

No matter which squats you do, always keep a neutral spine to avoid rounding your back, do not lean forward or cave in your knees.

Standing Crunch

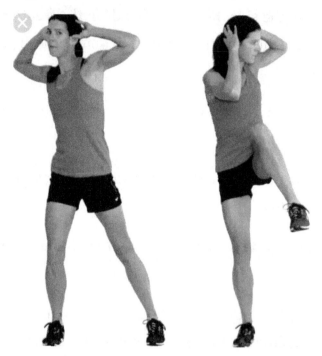

Standing crunch is like a sit-up exercise, only that instead of lying down, you perform it while standing. This exercise aims at strengthening the core, the glute, and other lower back muscles and, you do not require any equipment to perform it.

How to do it

- Stand on your mat with your feet hip-width apart, knees slightly bent, shoulders in line with your hips, and head in its neutral position.

- Interlock your fingers at the back of your head and tuck your chin.

- Engage the core by tucking your pelvis and pulling down your ribs.

- Evenly distribute your weight on your feet, bend your right knee and push your right leg up.

- Tighten your abs, then push your left elbow and shoulder towards your right leg until the elbow almost touches the knee.

- Stay in this position for a second or 2, then slowly lower your leg and push your shoulders up to return to the starting position. Remember to keep a tight core.

- Repeat the above moves with your left leg and right elbow.

- Continue this exercise, alternating sides for at least 10 minutes.

If you have a pre-existing back problem or are recovering from an injury, consult with your doctor if it is safe for you to perform a standing crunch. Also, focus on how your body feels with every crunch. If you experience any discomfort or pain, stop the exercise immediately and take a break before moving on to the next exercise.

Tree Pose Exercise

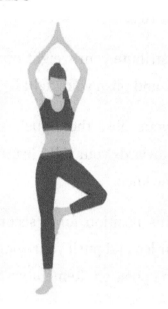

Also called the Vrksasana exercise, the tree pose exercise aims at improving balance, concentration and relaxation. It is an easy-to-do pose, making it an ideal exercise for people of all age groups.

How to do it

- Stand straight on your mat with your feet touching and hands stretched on your sides.

- Bend your elbows and bring your palms together in front of you.

- Take a few deep breathes and focus your gaze and attention on an object or place of choice in front of you.

- Bend your right knee and lift your right leg such that its sole is inside your left thigh and its toes are pointing to the ground. Slowly keep lifting your right leg until its sole is against your left knee or thigh. To maintain your balance, slightly move your weight to your straight leg.

- Extend your arms upwards such that your palms are touching on top of your head, forming an upside-down 'V.' If your arms cannot touch, raise them as high as you can.

- Hold this position for a minute.

- Slowly return to the starting position.

- Repeat the above moves with your left sole against your right knee or thigh.

- Continue this exercise for 10 minutes, alternating sides.

If you find it hard to hold the sole of the raised foot in place, fold a small towel or a small mat and put it between your inner knee/thigh and your sole.

If you have weak knees, you can start by practicing the tree pose exercise while lying on a mat, then slowly advance to a standing position by reducing the "pausing time" to 5 or 10 seconds, then increasing it (pausing time) as your knees gain strength. Also, you can start by lifting your foot a few inches off the floor then advance to the full tree pose exercise. If need be, perform this exercise with a chair or a table in front of you for support.

If you have lower back issues, start by performing this exercise against a wall before trying it without support.

To modify the tree pose exercise, increase the "pausing time" for each leg and try to close your eyes throughout the exercise.

Lunge Exercises

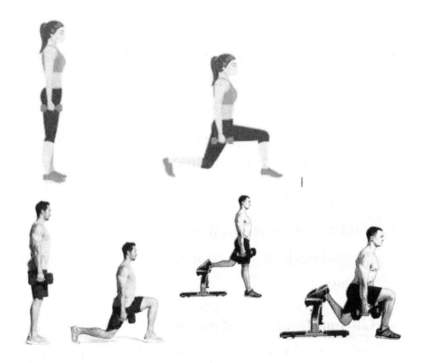

The lunge is an exercise that will help improve your lower body strength by working on your calves, glutes, quadriceps, and hamstrings. It also works on your lower back muscles and abdominal muscles. Different types of lunge exercises will help boost your balance during different daily activities, e.g., when changing direction or motion, preventing you from falling.

How to do it

- To perform the basic lunge, stand on your mat with your arms on your waist.

- Place your right foot about a foot in front of your left foot and relax your shoulders and back.

- Engage your core and bend your legs such that your front knee is in line with your toes and the front thigh is parallel to the floor. Your back knee should be a few inches off the ground. Let your front leg carry most of your weight and support and balance your body using your back leg.

- Hold this position for a second or two and avoid any temptation to lean forward or bend your front knee further.

- Lift your front leg and use your back leg for support to return to the starting position. Makes sure to push through your heels to ensure you can fully engage your glute muscles.

- Repeat this move for a minute.

- Switch sides such that your left foot is in front and perform the above exercise for a minute.

- Continue doing this exercise for 10 minutes, alternating sides after every 1 minute, and keep your neck relaxed and your head still.

The good news is that you do not have to worry if you cannot bend your front foot to 90 degrees or lower your back foot to almost touching the ground. Just lower yourself as low as you can. You will still improve your balance without straining your knee joints.

Some lunge variations you can try are:

Walking Lunge

To perform this exercise, look for a large space that will allow you to take 10 -15 big steps. Start by doing a few basic lunges and when you are in a lunge position, instead of pushing through your heels to return to a standing position, push your back leg forward (perhaps your right leg) such that it now is the front leg and bend its knee to get into a lunging position. Keep your right leg (now the back leg) in position for support as you perform this move. Continue this exercise (where you will seem to be "walking" forward) for 15 repetitions. Turn around and start to perform a walking lunge to the starting spot, with the other leg taking the lead (in this case, your left leg).

Lunge with Torso Rotation

To perform this lunge modification, start by doing some basic lunges; then, when you are in a lunging position (with your left leg in front) and feeling stable, rotate your torso to the left using your core. Hold this position for a few seconds, rotate your torso back to the center, and return to the starting position. Repeat this move with your right leg in front and your torso rotated to the right. Continue doing the lunge with torso rotation for 10 minutes.

Reverse Lunge

The reverse lunge is different from the basic lunge in that instead of taking a step forward, you will be taking a step backward, but of the same width as you do when performing basic lunges. Also, you will be using your back leg to carry your weight and your front leg for support, stability, and balance (the vice versa of basic lunge).

Elevated Foot Lunge

To perform elevated foot lunge, either put your front foot (front foot elevated lunge) or rear foot (rear foot elevated lunge) on a step or a bench and then perform basic lunge while in that position. You can also perform front elevated foot lunge with an Olympic lifting bumper plate or use an exercise ball to do rear elevated foot lunge. When performing elevated foot lunges, avoid the urge to bend your front knee past your toes or to collapse your back knee inwards.

Lunges with Weights

When you are confident that your balance is good and are up for a challenge, try to add weights to any of the above lunges. For example, you can hold dumbbells in each hand and straighten them on your sides, place a barbell on top of your shoulders or hold a kettlebell, a barbell, or a plate over your head with your arms locked out and in line with your ears.

However, start with small weights, then advance to heavier weights, depending on your performance. If possible, have a trainer, a coach, or a friend who has lunge knowledge to ensure you perform them correctly with weights to avoid injuring yourself or tearing your muscles.

One thing you need to know about lunging is that stepping too far can affect the flexibility of the rear leg, making you unstable. On the other hand, stepping too close will put too much pressure on your knees and could lead to joint pains.

To avoid this, measure your stance by lowering your rear knee to the ground while in a lunge position, then adjusting your stance until both knees are at a 90 degrees angle.

Plank Exercise

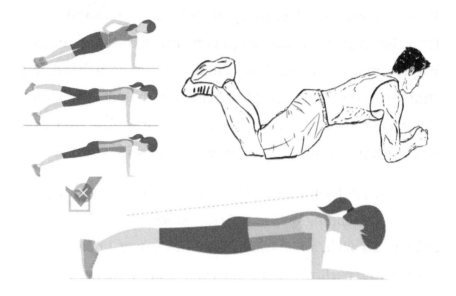

Plank is another exercise that can help improve your balance as it works on the core, connecting the upper and lower body parts. A strong core translates into a strong spine, which leads to improved balance.

The other muscles targeted by planks are the glute, shoulder, leg, and arm muscles. Essentially, plank exercise engages almost every part of the body; hence, including it in your workout routine will lead to more than one benefit.

How to do it

To perform basic/standards plank exercise:

- While on your mat, get into a horizontal position with your face facing down and hands under your shoulders or a bit wider. Your fingers should be pointing forward, and your palms should press down on the mat.

- Keep your feet hip-width apart, let your toes be on the floor for support, and increase your stability by squeezing your glute muscles.

- Tighten your core muscles and keep your gaze not more than a foot away from your hands to ensure you can maintain a neutral neck and spine. Keep your head, neck, back, butt, and hips in line, i.e., do not let them sink or creep up.

- Hold this position for around 30 seconds before releasing but do not hold your breath; instead, keep a normal breathing pattern.

- Continue for 10 repetitions.

- For every session you perform this exercise, increase the "holding time" by 20 or more seconds, depending on how comfortable each plank feels.

Some plank variations you can try to simplify or make your plank exercise more challenging are:

Forearm Plank

For seniors or people recovering from an injury, forearm planks are one of the best plank variations you can start with before advancing to standard or more challenging plank exercises.

This exercise differs from the basic plank in that instead of using your palms for support, you will place your elbows on the floor (at shoulder-width apart) with your forearm lying on the ground.

Remember to keep your spine in its natural curvature, tighten your core and maintain a straight posture from head to heels. For forearm planks, start by holding for a minute, then gradually increase your "holding time."

Knee Plank

For knee plank, instead of straightening your legs and supporting yourself with your toes, kneel without putting stress on your back and support your upper back with either your elbows or palms.

Keep your abs tight throughout the exercise but do not slack your back. Lift your legs off the ground while performing this exercise and hold for a minute or two.

Side Plank

- On your mat, lie on your right side with your legs straight and feet touching.

- Engage your core and use your right elbow or right palm to prop your body up as you push your hips off the ground.

- Keep your feet, hips and knees stacked and continue raising your body until you form a straight line from your heels to your shoulders.

- Hold your 30-60 seconds and then return to the starting position.

- Switch sides such that you are lying on your left side and repeat the above steps.

- Continue for 10 minutes, alternating sides.

You can add a challenge to the side plank exercise by lifting the arm or leg (or both) that is not supporting you toward the ceiling such that your body forms a "T" shape.

Plank with Elbow Lift

- Start in a basic plank position with your body in a straight line from heels to shoulders.

- As you squeeze your upper back muscles and engage your core, push your right elbow back.

- Keep your hand close to your body and place your palm on your right rib cage.

- Hold for a second or 2, then return your hand to the starting position.

- Repeat the above moves with your left elbow.

- Continue this exercise for a minute or so, alternating sides.

One-Legged Plank

As the name suggests, this plank variation exercise requires you to get into a basic or forearm plank position then lift one leg at a time. When lifting your leg, keep your back straight and hips parallel to the ground.

When performing any type of plank, do not hold your breath. It might feel like the natural thing to do, but it is not. Not supplying your body with oxygen may lead to undesired results like nausea, muscle injury, or dizziness.

Also, always keep your neck and head in a neutral position by keeping your gaze a few inches in front of your elbows or fingers (depending on the type of plank you are performing).

Lastly, to ensure you engage your core and glute muscles to the maximum, do not push your butt upwards to the ceiling or downwards to the ground. Instead, aim to keep your upper body in a proper position, i.e., forming a straight line, which will translate into a neutral butt position. These two positions will allow you to get the best results on your glute and core muscles.

Sit and Stand Exercise

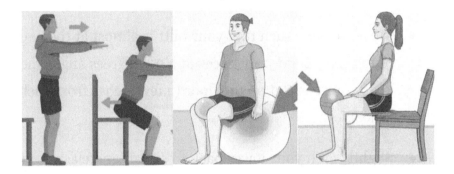

Almost all activities we do every day involve the sitting and standing motion, which can lead to a fall when done wrongly.

The Sit and stand exercise helps strengthen the core, lower back, and leg muscles, improving balance and stability. The good thing about this exercise is that you can incorporate it into your life by mindfully doing it every time you stand from a sitting position.

How to do it

- Sit on a sturdy and standard height chair, which you can comfortably position your feet on the ground. Ensure the chair won't roll or slide on the floor by putting it on an exercise mat or against a wall. If you have pre-existing balance or back pain issues, perform this exercise with a sturdy surface in front of you, e.g., a table or a countertop for the support you will need if you lose balance when standing.

- Move forward such that your butt is almost at the end of the seat. Bend your knees at a 90 degrees angle and keep your feet flat on the floor (a few inches from each other).

- Slightly arch your lower back to sit tall and clasp your hands behind your head (if you don't have balance challenges) or, hold them together in front of your chest or straighten them in front of you (if you feel like you might want to reach out for support).

- Without moving your feet, lean forward, squeeze your glute muscles, engage your leg muscles and slowly push yourself up to a standing position. Remember to keep your spine in its natural curvature. If you find it hard to push yourself up, push through your hands by placing them on the seat or arms of your chair.

However, try as much as possible to perform this exercise without the help of your hands.

- Slowly lower yourself back to the starting position.

- Do this exercise 10 times (1 set), take a short break, then complete another 2 sets.

After mastering the sit and stand exercise, you can include a challenge in your exercise routine by:

Doing More Repetitions

You can modify the sit and stand exercise by increasing the number of repetitions you perform in each set to 15 or 20 to make it more intense.

Putting an Object between Your Knees

If you find it hard to keep your knees at a 90 degrees angle, you can modify your sit and stand exercise by placing a small object between your knees and squeezing it with your legs as you stand. Examples of objects you can use are a small exercise ball, stuffed animals, a small pillow, a book, or a yoga block. Sitting and standing with any of these objects in place will help engage your leg and butt muscles.

Using an Exercise Ball

Instead of sitting on a chair, try doing this exercise while sitting on an exercise ball. This will add a challenge to your exercise as it will be harder to stand from an exercise balance, hence better results in toning your core and strengthening your leg and glute muscles.

You can also try putting an object between your legs when performing the sit and stand exercise on an exercise ball for a challenge.

Using Weights

You can boost the intensity of the sit and stand exercise by adding weights, e.g., dumbbells. To do this variation, hold dumbbells with your elbows bent and palms in front of your chest or hands stretched out in front of you, and then follow the steps for doing the standard sit and stand exercise. It's best to start will small weights (e.g., 1.4 kg or 2.3 kg weights), then gradually move to heavier weights once you can comfortably do 3 sets of 20 repetitions.

Single-Leg Stand Exercise

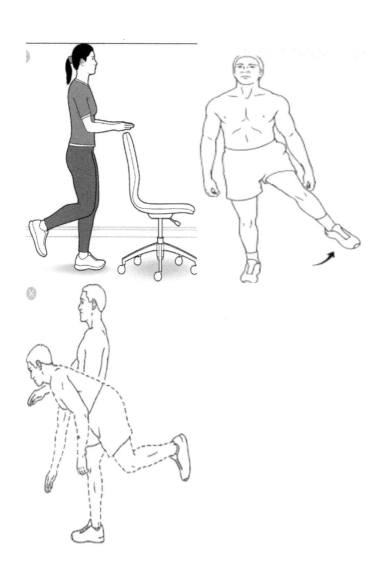

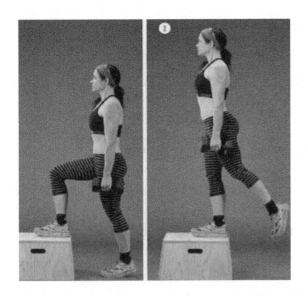

Normally, most people have one stronger and more coordinated leg, which can lead to imbalance. Adding single-leg exercise (one leg exercise) to your workout routine will help correct this condition, improving your balance and strength — it targets your glute muscles, leg muscles, core muscles, hip flexors, and abductors.

How to do it

Start by practicing the basic single-leg exercise with support through the following steps:

- Stand on your exercise mat with a seat or wall in front of you such that only your fingertips touch the seat or wall when you stretch out your hands. Keep your legs at shoulder-width apart.

- Let your fingertips hold the seat or touch the wall as you bend your right knee such that your right leg's toes are pointing downward behind you. Keep your spine in its natural curvature.

- Hold this position for 10 to 20 seconds.

- Slowly return your right leg to the starting position.

- Switch sides and repeat the above steps with your left leg lifted.

- Continue this exercise, switching sides until you complete 3 repetitions.

After mastering this exercise, you can modify it by:

Doing It without Support

Move away from the wall or chair and practice the above steps with your palms at your hips, hands stretched out in front of you but not touching anything, or hands extended on your sides.

Adding Hip Flexion

To perform this variation, stand on one leg and push the other leg up toward your chest such that its thigh is parallel to the ground, then gently return it to the starting position. Do 3 reps on each side. You can slightly bend your straight leg at the knee to increase your stability.

You can modify single-leg exercise with hip flexion by rotating the lifted leg (from side to side). This will introduce a challenge to the strength of your hip muscles.

Also, you can move your head up and down or rotate it from side to side when standing on one leg- with hip flexion to increase the intensity of your exercise.

Flexing Your Trunk

After bending your leg backward (say your left leg), lean your chest forward until your right hand's fingertips are touching the ground. Hold this position for 10 to 20 seconds, then slowly return to the starting position. Switch legs and repeat. Continue doing this exercise until you complete 3 sets on each leg. Throughout the exercise, keep your lifted leg bent and your back straight.

Swinging Your Leg

Perform a few reps of the basic single-leg exercise, then start swinging your lifted leg forward and backward or laterally in a controlled manner for a minute, then switch sides.

Doing Single Leg with Step-Up

Stand upright with a high step or bench in front of you. Contract your glute muscles as you step on the bench with your left leg and push your right leg backward. Hold for a second or 2, then lower your right leg until it touches the ground. Continue raising and suspending your right leg for 20 seconds, switch sides, and repeat until you complete 3 sets on each side.

Doing Single-Leg Exercise with Squat and Twist

While standing on one leg, extend your hands in front of you and move your trunk forward, keeping your back straight. Lower yourself into a squat, keep your bend leg in its position, and twist your upper body to the opposite side, i.e., if you are standing on your right leg, twist your upper body to the left. Hold for 30 seconds, return to the starting position and repeat for a minute or 2. Switch legs and continue for another 1 or 2 minutes.

Doing One-Leg Exercise with Weights

You can try increasing the intensity by including 0.5lb dumbbells or medicine balls to your one-leg exercises. For example, you can hold these weights with your hands on your sides, stretched out in front of you or over your head in any of the above variations.

Bridge Exercise

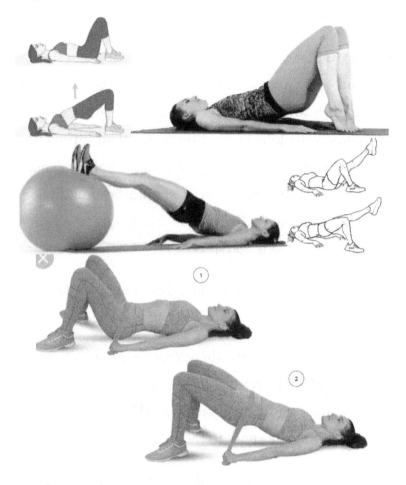

The Bridge exercise —also called glute-bridge or hip raise— is another exercise that improves balance by working on the glute, core, hamstrings, and leg muscles. People of all ages can perform this exercise because of its different variations. But before we look at these simpler or harder modifications of the bridge exercise, you have to learn how to do the standard or basic one.

How to do it

- Onto your mat, lie on your back with knees bent at 90 degrees angle and feet flat on the ground (directly below your knees), slightly wider than hip-width. Let your toes be at 45 degrees angle pointing outward (meaning that your knees should be pointing in the same direction). Keep your hands stretched on your sides along your body.

- Squeeze and tighten your glute and core muscles by pressing your lower back on the mat slightly.

- Press your feet onto the ground and push your pelvis up until you are suspended off the ground by your shoulders and feet. Your body should be in a straight line from your knees to the chin.

- Keep your core squeezed and glute muscles tight (pull your butt towards your lower back but do not arch your spine).

- Stay in this position for 30 seconds.

- Slowly lower your hips and pelvis to get to the starting position.

- Continue doing this exercise for 5 to 10 minutes.

After mastering the basic bridge exercise, you can spice up your workout sessions by trying the following variations:

Bridge Exercise with Toes Pointing Forward

This exercise is not that different from the basic bridge exercise; the primary difference is that you have to adjust your feet to hip-width and keep your toes pointing forward. As a result, your knees will be closer to each other, improving access to your midline glute muscles and inner thigh muscles. Remember to keep your knees above your toes.

Bridge Exercise with Heels Raise

Lie on your exercise mat as if you are performing a basic bridge with toes pointing forward, and as you push your pelvis off the ground, raise your heels off the ground too. Hold this position for a few seconds, then slowly lower your pelvis to the starting position, keeping your heels off the ground. Continue doing this exercise for 5 to 10 minutes.

Bridge Exercise with Toes Raise

This exercise is similar to bridge exercise with heel raises; however, instead of pushing your heels off the ground, you will be raising toes.

One-Leg Bridge Exercise

Lie on your back with your feet flat on the ground, hands at your sides, and knees bent. As you push your pelvis off the ground, raise your right foot until it's straight and pointing to the ceiling. Keep your hips firm as you hold this position for 30 seconds. Slowly lower your pelvis back to the starting position. Continue this exercise with your right foot up for 5 minutes, then switch sides. Continue doing this exercise with your left foot up for another 5 minutes.

You can also modify the one-leg bridge exercise by keeping your pelvis in the air and lowering your raised leg instead.

Bridge Exercise with Medicine Ball (Elevated Bridge)

This exercise is quite a challenge but is a great variation for boosting stability. To do the elevated bridge, get into the starting position of a standard bridge exercise and place your feet on a medicine ball or stability ball. Drive through your legs and push your hips and pelvis off the floor to get into a bridge position. Stay in this position for a minute or 2 and return to the starting position.

Bridge Exercise with Weights or Resistance Bands

Put a weight on your hips and hold it with your hands to keep it from falling, then perform a basic bridge exercise.

For variation with bands, place a hip circle, a resistance band, or a loop a few inches above your knees and then follow the steps for doing a basic bridge exercise. You can also modify this exercise by placing a hip circle, loop, resistance band, or a tube above your knees hips and holding it down to the floor with your wrists on both sides. Ensure the band stays on the floor as you perform the standard bridge exercise.

These variations engage the glute core and hip muscles at a higher level due to the resistance brought by the weights or the bands.

When performing bridge exercises (it doesn't matter the variation), always keep your core squeezed and glute muscles tight to get the best results.

Do not raise your hips too high such that your back arches, which can lead to back injuries or straining. Also, do not let your hips sag, as this can lead to injuries too. To avoid these, always keep your body in a straight line from shoulders through your abdomen to your knees. During your first few bridge exercise sessions, you can build up your core, glute, and thigh muscles strength by staying in the bridge position for 5 seconds as you then advance to full range motion.

At the end of these balance exercise sessions, you will feel fatigued. As a result, it is important to set some time for cool-down exercises, which will help make you feel relaxed.

Let us look at other reasons why cool-down exercises are important and some examples you can include in your balance exercise routine.

Chapter 4: Cool-down Exercise/Stretches

It is very tempting to skip the cool-down part of your exercise routine, maybe because you feel exhausted or running out of time, but do not skip the cool-down. Cool-down stretches will help start your journey to recovery and make you feel relaxed through the following ways:

- Cooling down will lower your blood pressure, body temperature, and heartbeat back to normal, making you ready to go on with other daily activities.

- Cool-down stretches will help reduce lactic acid production in the body, reducing stiffness and muscles cramps.

- Stretching after the working-out will prevent your blood from pooling, a situation that can leave you feeling dizzy or light-headed.

Due to these and many more benefits, you need to plan for at least 10 minutes for cool-down exercises.

Some of the stretches you can try are:

Corpse Pose

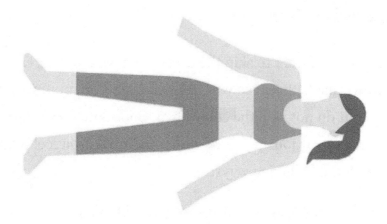

How to do it

- Onto your mat, lie on your back with your hands on your sides along your body, legs straight and feet wider than hip-width. Keep your palms facing the ceiling and your toes pointing outward.

- Take a deep breath in and out and let your body lie heavily on the mat.

- Release any tension and tightness in your muscles to relax your body.

- Lie in this position for 5 minutes or more until your body feels fully relaxed.

Standing Forward Bend Exercise

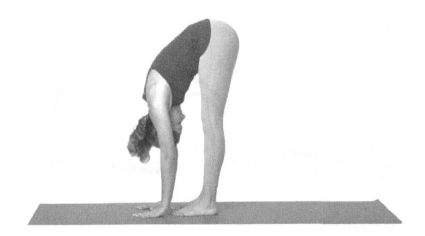

How to do it

- Stand tall on your exercise mat with your feet at hip-width and hands stretched out on your sides along your body.

- Hinge your hips, slightly bend your knees and push your upper body forward.

- Extend your spine and stretch your hands until your palms are touching the floor. If this seems challenging, put your hands on a block in front of you or interlock your fingers behind your head. Let your head sink toward the floor.

- Stay in this position for 30 seconds.

- Slowly return to the starting position.

- Continue doing this stretch for 5 minutes.

Child's Pose Exercise

How to do it

- Onto your mat, get into a table-top position.

- Lower your hips and bend your knees to sit on your heels.

- Let your chest rest on your thighs with your forehead on the mat.

- Stretch out your arms in front of you, keeping your palms on the mat.

- Stay in this position for 3 to 5 minutes, and remember to keep breathing to let oxygen into your body, relaxing your muscles.

- Return to starting position.

Seated Forward Bend

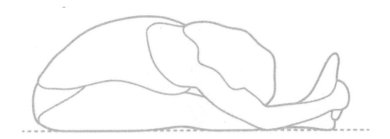

How to do it

- Onto your exercise mat, sit with your hands on your sides or lap and legs straight in front of you.

- Lean forward with your upper body and place your hands on the floor beside your legs or hold your feet.

- Keep leaning until your chest is touching or almost touching your thighs.

- Stay in this position for 3 to 5 minutes. Remember to keep breathing in a controlled manner.

Cow/Cat Stretch

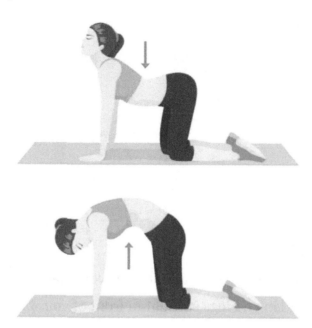

How to do it

- Onto your exercise mat, get on your knees and hands. Keep your hands in line with your shoulders and your knees in line with your hips.

- Take a deep breath in and slowly arch your back as you lift your head to look to the ceiling. This is the "cow" position

- As you breathe out, slowly round your back and let your head drop towards the mat. This is the cat position

- Continue doing this cow and cat sequence for 3 to 5 minutes.

Figure 4 Stretch

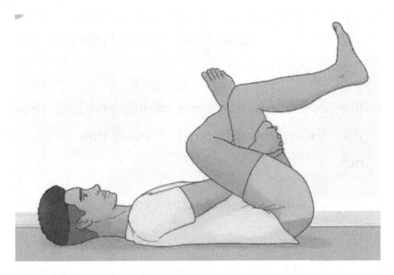

Figure 4 stretch exercise will help release your glute muscles and open up your hip muscles for recovery.

How to do it

- Onto your exercise mat, lie on your back with feet flat on the ground (hip-width apart) and knees bent at a 90 degrees angle.

- Lift your right leg and place it on top of your left leg such that your right ankle is on your left knee.

- Interlock your fingers at the back of your left thigh and pull toward your face. Keep your trunk and back pressed against the floor.

- Draw your left thigh as close to your face as possible, and press your right elbow on your right knee to push it away from you.

- Stay in this position for a minute and keep drawing your left leg toward your face every time you breathe out.

- Release your thigh and return your legs to the starting position.

- Switch sides and repeat the above steps with your left ankle on your right knee.

- Continue doing this stretch for 5 minutes, alternating sides.

Legs-Up the Wall Pose

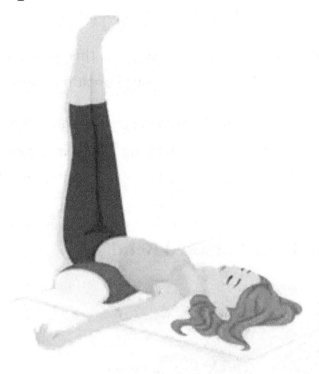

How to do it

- Put your exercise mat next to a wall and lie on your back with your butt a few inches away from the wall but keep your tailbone on the mat. This position should leave your head and back at a right angle with the wall.

- Let your hands lie on your stomach, overhead, or your sides along your body.

- Extend your legs up the wall. Relax your knees and keep your feet parallel to the ground.

- Relax your body and stay in this position for 3 minutes. Maintain a controlled breathing pattern.

- Slowly return to the starting position and sit for about 30 seconds before standing. This is necessary as rapidly coming out of an inverted position can lead to dizziness that causes a fall.

Head to Knee Forward Bend

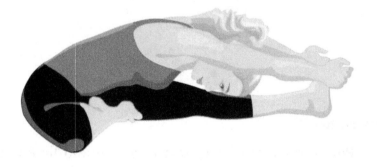

How to do it

- Sit on your mat and extend your left leg. Bend your right knee and push the sole inward such that it's pressing on the inner thigh of your right leg.

- Raise your hands and align your sternum with the inside of the extended leg.

- Use your hips to pivot yourself as you lean forward such that your hands are touching the sole of your left leg and your head is on your left knee.

- Hold this position for a minute.

- Return to the starting position, then switch sides.

- Continue doing head to knee forward bend for 6 minutes, switching sides.

Reclining Twist Stretch

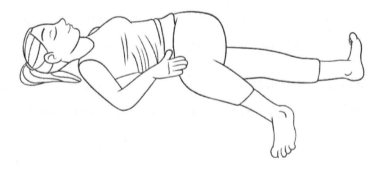

The reclining twist is a good cool-down stretch that will help release your lower back.

How to do it

- Lie on your back and bend your knees on your mat, keeping your feet flat on the ground. You can place a pillow under your head for support; let your hand lie on your sides along your body.

- Draw your knees toward your chest then, extend your right leg to lie on the floor.

- Take a deep breath in and continue pushing your left leg up.

- Stretch your left arm to the left until it is at the same height as your shoulders. Keep your left palm facing down.

- Slightly move your hips to the left and place your right palm on your left knee.

- Let your left knee drop to your right side as you breathe out. Keep your right hand in place.

- Shift your head to the left and keep a soft gaze on your left fingertips. Relax your shoulders such that they press onto your mat with no tension.

- Relax your knees and toes and let them drop to the ground.

- Hold this position for 2 minutes, take a deep breath, and slowly return to the starting position.

- Repeat the other side with your left leg straight on the floor.

- Continue doing this exercise for 8 minutes, i.e., two times on each side.

- When you are in the starting position, pull your knees toward your chest with your hand, hold this position for a few seconds, extend your legs on the mat and slowly get to a standing position.

After you cool down, you can continue with your day's activities without the fear of falling.

Conclusion

It is never too late to regain your strength and courage, and it is never too early to start working on your balance and stability. Make it your goal to have at least 3 (30- 45 minutes) balance exercise sessions every week and wait to see how they will transform your life.

You will be able to proudly walk into any room without the fear of falling or the need for a walking stick.

On top of that, you will have a fit and healthy body because, as stated early, balance exercises target different muscle groups. Imagine being in your old age with people your age or younger than you wishing they had the balance and stability you have. How great would that feel?

Lucky for you, balance exercises are easy to do, meaning you don't have to sign up for a gym membership: you do them at home. All you have to do is check your schedule, create time for balance exercises, order your exercise mat, go buy some comfortable workout clothes and shoes, and get right to it.

PS: I'd like your feedback. If you are happy with this book, please leave a review on Amazon.

Please leave a review for this book on Amazon by visiting the page below:

https://amzn.to/2VMR5qr

Made in the USA
Middletown, DE
24 April 2022